If Walls Could Talk

If Walls Could Talk

Don't Let Epilepsy control you!

Ann Marie Gillie

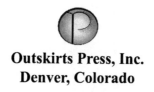

Outskirts Press, Inc.
Denver, Colorado

To all my boys
and
Jill

Outskirts Press, Inc.
http://www.outskirtspress.com

ISBN: 978-1-4327-5087-9

Outskirts Press and the "OP" logo are trademarks belonging to Outskirts Press, Inc.

PRINTED IN THE UNITED STATES OF AMERICA

Table of Contents

EPILEPSY

My personal definition on the word…..

E   *Empowering*

P   *Persuasive*

I   *Idle* (is where we seem to be at times)

L   *Learning experience*

E   *Enduring*

P   *Positive* (when you decide to see it that way)

S   *Safety* (should always come first)

Y   *Yield* (but don't ever stop)

If Walls Could Talk

By: Ann Marie Gillie

They see us from all angles
Every step we take
Sleeping, talking, cleaning house
Even times we ache
They catch us sneaking cookies
Or kissing in the dark
They help us hang our pictures
And let us decorate them with art
We sometimes rough them up a bit
Even color them real bright
Punch holes and add new windows
To make an old room a new sight
If only they could tell us
The things that they have seen
A wall could write a million books
I wonder if they dream
So as you walk around your home
And gaze at your walls
Remember if a wall could talk
The fun could end for all

I wrote this several months after my surgery and would like
to dedicate it to anyone and everyone that lives with or knows
someone with Epilepsy!

I have been putting together a story about my life with epilepsy since my surgery, which was back in December 2002. I think the writing has been more of a "personal therapy session" than anything; nevertheless, it has helped me in many ways! For my self, having epilepsy was definitely a learning experience, as well; it was like being on a roller coaster, going around and around and around, it seemed endless. I know that epilepsy comes with positives and negatives, but it all depends on how you handle it. Personally, I hate how society has put a brand on those with seizures or epilepsy, as if they are individuals that can't make it in life, are incompetent and can't function in the "real world". Well let me tell you, I went over 20 years being on meds and having all kinds of seizures, did that stop me? Hell no!

I finished high school, college, have had three children and never stopped doing things that I wanted to do and not just because I am stubborn either. I never let epilepsy control me! I am not a physician, psychiatrist, or neurosurgeon, I am just someone who feels the need to put my ideas and thoughts on paper, I am a survivor and you can be to. Even if your seizures don't come to an end like mine did, you need to stay positive and remember you are not alone, work around what you can do not what you can't do. Yes my life has been through some major adjustments, but in the big picture, I am where I should be. I am married and have three very active boys, Mathew, Cameron and our newest addition to the family, Nathan, I work, volunteer and live life to the fullest! The oldest two have seen me at my worst, which is something I wish I could erase from their memories, but than I think, that life isn't always about smiles and happy times, it is about dealing with problems and working things out together as a family.

I have listened to some pretty interesting motivational speakers in the past few years and I have to give credit to some of them, because if it weren't for me hearing what they accomplished, struggled with and set forth to do in their own lives, I may not of decided to do what I am striving for and that is reaching out to you. Letting you know that it is alright, life can go still go on when you have epilepsy and the choices you make are ones that can affect you for the rest of your life. So sit back and take a deep breath, and know that your life is what you make of it! In this book I talk about my history with seizures, my surgery and the dark recovery I had, which did have light at the end, thankfully. As well I have included some facts, history, and comments from my on-line support group and much more, you may just have to keep reading to see.

1

What is Epilepsy and its Triggers

After all I have been through, I still think I lead a pretty normal life, I work, volunteer and up until my surgery was involved in sports, which I have been gradually getting back into. I think I might just hold back on the boxing though, but you never know, I have always been a pretty stubborn individual and has never really liked being told I can't do something. Now, I originally started this story in 2003, thinking I would be done with it that maybe it was just a form of therapy that I needed, but as more time went by and I dealt with different aspects of the recovery process and needed to continue with it. I already had a rough copy typed up, but when I read it, I was amazed how I wrote. My sentences were very simple and short; the words I used were only one and two syllables, so I thought that if I could just sit back down in front of the computer and rewrite my story that it would give me some closure on the whole ordeal, but it is definitely not something I want to forget. So that is why I am typing here today! There were days were I would sit back and think "why me?" Than I think of disasters like 9/11, the fighting and killing that continues in the world today and people dying of hunger, aids, you name it. So is what I have to say really that important? Damn right it is! Epilepsy was not something I asked for, or that my parents wished upon me, it was unfortunately something that I as a person was meant to deal with. Many people get very confused with the whole concept of Epilepsy and Seizures, they really don't know what it is, what is does to a person or what causes it (in most cases). **Epilepsy is a physical condition characterized by sudden and brief changes in how the brain works.** It is a **DISORDER** not a **DISEASE**, like many people refer to it as.

Did you know that approximately 6 % of Canadians have epilepsy and that an average of 42 people a day in Canada learn that they have the disorder? Well they do! Just because a person has one seizure does not mean they have epilepsy! Approx 10% of the world population will have one seizure during their lifetimes. To be diagnosed with or to say a person has epilepsy is defined by a person having **two or more** unprovoked seizures. It has been documented to that epilepsy is one of the worlds oldest recognized conditions, it is misunderstood, discriminated against and has had a lot of social stigma for centuries now towards it. Some of the stigma around the world definitely impacts the quality of life for people with the disorder as well as their families. It is said that approx 50 million people in the world have epilepsy! A lot of people don't know the exact causes of seizures, there are many different triggers, but some of the main ones are:

- Stress(which a lot of people say they don't have)
- Missed Medication(which a lot of people have done)
- Poor Nutrition
- Lack of Sleep
- Flickering of Lights

- Emotions(anger, fear and worry)
- Illness
- Skipping Meals
- Heat and Humidity

Even on the boys electronic or computer games, there are warnings for people with seizures, they think that just means more play time for them, little do they know, I love to play too, I actually have a wicked golf score on the Tiger Woods X - Box game, I just wish I could golf like that when I am "actually" golfing on a real course. Today, there are several forms of therapy for seizures; the major form of treatment is long-term drug therapy, which has always been what I had personally gone with. However, as I got older, I seemed to be very open to other forms of therapy and treatment, I have never been afraid to try new things! If surgery did not come around for me as an option I think I would of tried just about anything and I mean anything!

2

How it all began for me

It all started for me in 1972. I really don't recall much from my early years having seizures, but I have been told enough stories from family that I feel like I do. Apparently, it was horrible, devastating and not something you wish upon anyone. My parents said that seeing me go into a grand mal seizure at 2 years old was heartbreaking, mostly because, there was nothing they could do, or they didn't know what to do. My seizures all started because of a very high fever, my mom tells me that she had given me Aspirin before bedtime, as I was feeling quite warm, it seemed to work the times before she had used it on me, but not this one. My brother was woken that night by me crying, so he rushed into my parent's bedroom to wake them up and that is when it all started for me. I was taken to the nearest hospital in Toronto, where we were living and my parents were told that my temperature was getting higher and that is when the seizures began. I was put on medication (at 2 years old) to help control the seizures, it did work and it didn't. Before I started Nursery School I had suffered a severe seizure that left my right side paralyzed, being so young I don't recall any of it, but my family sure does. Dragging my right leg was how I would get around and my mom would have to do exercises with me daily to help strengthen my leg and arm. This was back in 1972, my parents were never told "why" my right side decided to go like it did, or why I was having both petit mal and grand mal seizures, an MRI was never done on me, not until I was in my 30's. My parents were also told that my right side would not stay paralyzed, that it would probably be a few weeks and the muscles and movement would go back to normal, but that I might not be right handed or have problems in the future with my right side. Well I remained paralyzed for about 6 months and to prove the doctors wrong, I did continue writing with my right hand and there was no limping. So everything seemed to be getting better; the seizures too were not as frequent and the medication seemed to be going alright as far as side effects.

I was on Phenobarb, three times a day and I have read that now it is a very popular drug at veterinary clinics, nice! There were a few times in elementary school that I scared my parents, in that, I would take short cuts home from school, which I knew not to, especially by myself. One day coming home from school, when I was in Gr.2, I decided to cut through the forest behind our apartment; this is when we were living in London, Ontario. Well I didn't make it all the way home. I don't recall the grand mal seizure, but I had one, and remained in the forest for quite a while before being found. Some high school kids were walking through and came across me shaking on the ground, so they wrapped me in their coat and carried me home. After that episode, I was told not to walk through the forest again by myself, I listened for a while, but that forest was the coolest short cut to school, our

5

amazing tree houses where in there and where we all hung out. At about 9 1/2 years old the seizures had seemed to stop, that is when I was weaned totally off the Phenobarb. Through the next 10 years I didn't have anything, no petit mals, grand mals or even an aura, I was seizure free, so I thought!

When I was 20 yrs old, on holidays in B.C with my mom, it was a nightmare. I had just gone for 10+ year's seizure free and drug free, but that was about to change. We were on Vancouver Island camping and my brain decided it was going to start the whole seizure ordeal over again, the seizures were back. I was devastated, wanted to hide in a small hole and not come out.

As soon as we got home, I went to see the doctor, went through all the testing and was immediately put back on pills. The seizures were petit mal, nevertheless, they were seizures. I would have two one day, than go a week with nothing, than one every second day for a while. I was so mad, irritated and extremely pissed off that they were back and going to change everything once again for me. I had my drivers license taken away, which was more upsetting than the seizures them selves, especially at 20 years old.

As time passed, the drugs seemed to be working fairly well; the seizures began to get less and less **once again**, I had to be seizure free for one year to be able to drive again and what a feeling that was when that time came. A few years went by, no seizures, no aura's, everything was good. I even became pregnant with our first son, Mathew, and I was still on medication. What did piss me off was that at 6 months pregnant the doctor decided to tell me what **ALL** the complications could be with taking anticonvulsan drugs and being pregnant. How nice of them at 6 months to tell me all that, I would rather have been told before or not tel me at all. I had dreams of horrible things happening to my baby (Mathew). I did continue taking my pills through the pregnancy, my dose was cut down slightly though. When Mathew was born, Dec 23, 1994, he had the ten toes, ten fingers, everything was good. I did go till Matt was 1 ½ years old before the seizures returned. I lost my Drivers License again; the dosage of my pills was put back up, it all seemed so repetitious!

Years later I decided one day, that I needed a second opinion, things were not getting any better and I felt I did not have the connection with my neurologist that I needed. I was always having my meds changed but never being tested to see if I could try something new. So I got a referral to see a new neurologist and he than had me in to see another neurologist at the University of Alberta Hospital in a couple months, where I was finally tested to see if surgery was an option. I had to stay in my room for 8 days with about 30 wires attached to my head; they were keeping track of the seizure patterns and seeing where exactly the seizures were coming from. During my testing I had enough seizures for them to be able to pin point where the seizures were coming from and from that I was told that I qualified for surgery. The only thing that kept me occupied in the room was having my husbands laptop to watch movies and also all my visitors, I hope they didn't mind my look; I probably looked like an octopus from mars. It was only four months after the testing that I did go in for surgery and I was more excited than a kid at Christmas time.

My test results from the MRI showed that my left hippocampus was small, irregular and increased signal compared to that of my right, which showed that I had mesial temporal sclerosis on the left, which is a specific pattern of hippocampal neuron cell loss and it might occur with other temporal lobe abnormalities (dual pathology). Mesial temporal sclerosis is the most common pathological abnormality in temporal lobe epilepsy. I still wish that an MRI would have been done on my back in the early 70's, maybe I would have lived a pretty normal life, at least minus the seizures. Here are a few pictures of me, one when I was five, me after my surgery and me now. I have no problem looking at the photo of me with all the staples in my head, because looking like that changed my life forever.

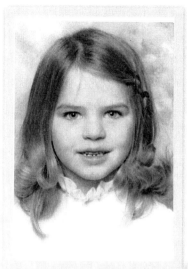

This is me, 5 years old, one of the high peaks of my seizures.

One week after my surgery....

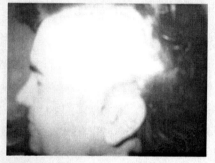

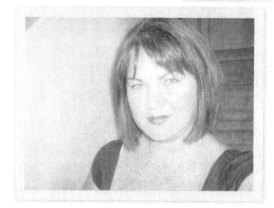

...and this is me today!

3

My Surgery   My Recovery

Well I have done a 180 deg turn, in that my life is finally at a place that I am happy and enjoying it. It has been just over 6 years since the surgery and I have been 110% seizure free ever since, knock on wood! I am so thankful to the surgeons and nurses at the University of Alberta Hospital for changing my life, they were all remarkable. The name of the surgery that I had was **Left Selective Amygdalohippocampectomy**, wow; say that five times really fast! When I was being wheeled down the hall at about 6:30 am at the U of A Hospital in Edmonton, it felt like the porter and I were the only ones in the building. It was so quiet; you could hear a pin drop, after taking lots of turns in the hallway and getting on the elevator we made it to the surgery area. "This was it", I thought, "I sure hope it works". I only had to wait for a while before transporting me right into the room, **WOW**.

I saw the tables along the back wall and it looked like there were a thousand instruments, tools and surgery utensils, so cool I thought. No, it didn't scare me at all, I love watching E.R, surgery or medical shows on TV, that stuff has never bothered me.

If it were up to me, I would have loved for my surgery to be tapped. Honestly. The bed I was lying on was than put next to the one where I was about to undergo some amazing work. I was lifted over to my new accommodations and was given a blanket to keep warm; these rooms never seem to be that comfy. I than had the anesthesiologist come over and introduce himself to me, I think he was a bit surprised that I was in such a good mood. Maybe most people having there skull cut open and brain drilled into don't usually have a smile on their face, I guess I am an exception.

After all the prepping and everyone making sure I was comfortable, it was time. I was told to take deep breaths and count when the mask was put over my face and that they would see me later that day. I just chuckled and asked if maybe they could do some touch up surgery while I was out, a little liposuction, tummy tuck, etc. I had a couple laughs and than told take a deep breath. I remember getting to 2 and after that, well I was out like a light. I honestly don't remember waking up after the surgery; my husband told me that he came into ICU to see me and I was in and out, not really responding to anything he was saying, I am sure I looked wonderful to. It was about a good 24 hours until I was awake enough to realize what was going on, I hadn't seen yet what I looked like or even really asked any questions. When I was finally able to get up off the bed, and very slowly, I headed for the bathroom, I wanted to see what they did. WOW. I had bandages all over my head.

As the bandages seemed to be a little loose, I gently tugged on one and it all came off, opp's, I said to the nurse. She new I was curious and told me she would help get them off. What a sight that was, 50 staples in the left side of my skull, and almost in the shape of a question mark. I asked why I couldn't feel anything and she said that I would be frozen for quite a while. So they just shaved the left side of my head for the surgery, not all of it, which was fine, I was able to trim down the other side and my hair grows like weeds do, so no worries there. After I was moved to a different room, from ICU, I had to work with a therapist on my walking. Apparently my brain was in neutral and I would almost have to say that I forgot how to walk. She had me do very slow laps around the hallways, I held on to the rails as tight as I could, it was very weird going from running up and down my stairs at home to being taught how to do it all over again. I worked with the therapist for about three or four days and after day six in the hospital I was sent home. I was told going home was the best way to recover. Following my surgery I had to attend quite a few sessions at the University Hospital to work on and improve my memory. Some of the testing seemed so tedious, it was like I was back in elementary school again counting to ten and having spelling tests. Some of the testing involved me being given 10 words, which were said out loud to me and than I would have to repeat them. I have to admit it sounds so easy, but my first couple of sessions was really tough; I maybe remembered 2 words out of the ten. I was also given an abstract picture to look at for 10 seconds and than had it taken away, I was supposed to draw it from memory; it was an interesting drawing to.

My surgery was called
Left Selective Amygdalohippocampectomy

Amygdala - An almond-shaped mass of gray matter in the anterior portion of the temporal lobe. Also called *amygdaloid nucleus*.

Hippocampus - is a neural structure in the medial temporal lobe.

Ectomy - excision, surgical removal.

Gradually I began to regain my memory skills and was done with my sessions, I did return for testing one year after the surgery and improved quite a bit. Now six years later I think I could honestly say that "I'm back". I never really lost my long term memory, just the short term. About 3 months after my surgery I picked up a pen and started writing poetry, I would have been the last person that you would ever think to write poems, but I love it! Of course it took some time to progress with my vocabulary, but I did with a bit of patience. My favorite poem to this day that I have written is, If Walls Could Talk, it was one that took me minutes to write, the words just seemed to come so smoothly and when I was finished writing it, I actually had shivers down my spine while reading it.

I have had several poems published and I am planning on continuing to write them. On top of writing, I also decided to try art. Now I know I am not an artist, but I try and to me that is all that matters. I think that I am a new person now with new ideas and I hope that with my experience I can help or reach out to at least one person who may be going through a similar experience, whether it is with epilepsy or not! Also, I have added in a few comments that I recently received from others around the world on my epilepsy support site and I have also put in my favorite poems and photos. It is really cool to talk with others that live 5000 km away but have had the same experiences as me. I also started a life after brain surgery support group on the internet and I am getting new members weekly, I love it. It is a great rush for me to be able to offer support to those who may feel they don't have any. Another interesting topic I have not mentioned yet is the opportunity I have been given to speak at several Epilepsy Forums. I have always been a person who "likes to talk" and for me to get up on stage and let it out, is a feeling that I would never want to loose. One Forum I spoke at was on 'Sex and Seizures" and the other was about "Living with epilepsy". I have added in a few comments from the **Sex and Seizures** forum for you to read as well. Both forums were very intriguing and powerful moments for me, as a person and as a speaker. I have also added in some epilepsy information that I felt would be helpful to those that may be looking for support, ideas or just general knowledge on epilepsy. I hope you enjoy the poems and please remember that a person with epilepsy is not someone to be afraid of or to feel awkward around, we (they) are people just like you and maybe just have a few glitches here and there, but doesn't everyone? Another great experience I was lucky to have had was when I went on television to talk about my experience with seizures, medications and of course my surgery. It was an experience of a lifetime!

Back in March 2006 I was on both Global TV and Breakfast Television in Edmonton, Alberta. I was a bit nervous at first, especially when getting ready in the back room, touching up my lipstick, making sure my hair looked alright, but overall I think I did pretty damn good. On both shows, it was funny the reaction I got from the hosts when I said the name of the surgery (Left Selective Amygdalohippocampectomy) and without error to, they both said "say that again". It definitely was a very positive and motivational experience for me and one that I would do again.

I also had the opportunity to be on Breakfast Television back in Sept 2002, I had a poem published in the book A Time of Trial

– Beyond the Terror of 9/11, 100% of the profit from the sales of the book went to the Red Cross relief fund for 9/11. While I was reading my poem out loud footage of the terrible disaster was being played, it was a very touching experience for me and one that left us all speechless after I was finished reading my poem. That is a moment that I felt privileged to be a part of and am honored that I was asked to be a part of. Luckily, I did not have a seizure while on TV, can you imagine if I did! Well let's not go there.

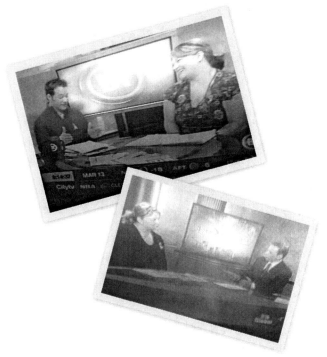

What an awesome experience I had being on two local tv stations to talk about my experince with seizures, my surgery and about Epilepsy Awareness Month.....March 2006

Thanks to Global Television and Breakfast television in Edmonton, Alberta!

In the summer of 2009 I started sending out emails to epilepsy organizations around the world and heard back from at least nine of them within the first week. I am looking to further expand my public speaking and hopefully take it internationally. I think that with all of my volunteering skills behind me and my dedication to volunteering with the Edmonton Epilepsy Association that I will gradually have more opportunities come my way. Some of my responses were ones that I was hoping to receive, in that I was put on their lists for upcoming events to assist as a speaker. Going for what I believe in and not giving up is a huge part of me! Quitting has never been an option.

One of the most touching things that did happen to me a couple nights before I went into the hospital for me surgery was having my doorbell ring, I was so surprised. Two moms from my son Mathews gr. 2 class had brought my family and I about 20 dinners, I didn't know what to say. There were boxes of fully cooked meals that the class parents had made, everything from pasta, chicken, casseroles, you name it. They told me (us) that the parents from the class got together to prepare meals for mostly Richard and the boys as they new I wouldn't be quite up to cooking right after my surgery. I was speechless, yes me speechless and that was one of the only times that I actually cried. I was so thankful to them. To me that was one event through this whole experience that will always stick with me, see there are still caring and nice people out there and I am happy to say I know them. Thanks.

4

My Depression After Surgery

Depression can be a very scary word for some people to say or even admit to having. I personally did fall in that category, the one of denial. Back when I was being tested to see if I even qualified for surgery I was told that depression is quite common after any type of neurosurgery, of course I didn't even take the time to research it or even think that I could ever be affected by it. After chatting with so many others on different epilepsy sites and on my support site on Facebook, depression seemed to be the #1 topic of conversation. It doesn't matter how old the person is, where they are from, whether it be the UK, USA, Canada, Australia etc, the majority of those who have had surgery for their seizures have all fallen into a major depression. The one very positive note that comes from this whole "depression" thing is that those going through this can see that they are not alone. We need to hear it from others, to be told, "hey, I know how you feel", "ya, I have been there to, it wasn't pleasant"; support, is to me the #1 thing that people need. I will say it a million time to, I wish I had a support group to fall back on when I was at my limit, at the edge of my plank, there probably was a group I just didn't look hard enough.

Not long after my surgery, I definitely was feeling different, very irritated, sad, moody, you name it and that was me. I had a hard time controlling my anger, especially at home, but not outside of the house so much. It was like I was a switch, I could turn on and off in the blink of an eye. Sitting in the tub, with the lights off for an hour or more was my way of escaping at times, but that wasn't me, I would normally be in and out in 5 minutes, as I have always had a hard time sitting still for to long.

Looking into depression and neurosurgery, I read a story on the studies of how many people with epilepsy have a mood disorder such as depression and it varied widely, ranging anywhere from 11 percent to 60 percent, which I found to be very interesting. In general, when standard methods are used, about 29 percent of people with epilepsy have a major depressive disorder. Research has also shown that people with epilepsy who are depressed often are not even diagnosed and about 50 percent of the time is never even treated for the problem. I did have the option to go on anti depressant medication when I felt this depression kicking in, but I refused to, I am thinking now that I probably should have, maybe it would of decreased my length of depression and the height that it even got to. In May 2003, 6 months after my surgery, my best friend Jill who I have known since I was 6 years old and who is a nurse in Florida, noticed a major change in my behaviour and mood. She told me, not asked me, to get down to there that I needed some away time to figure out what was going on inside my head. I had my husband and two sons at home and having them see what I was doing to myself and to them was not fare, so I went. I stayed with Jill for a week and did nothing but relax and have "**quiet time**", time to reflect on what I was going through and try to figure out, why? While in Florida I had a lot of time to myself as Jill was working and that gave me my days to try and figure out where to go from here. I spent hours down by the water and honestly I think that the peacefulness and sound of the water, birds and beautiful scenery around me helped me in a lot of ways. I actually relaxed and told myself "I can get through this".

Before going to Florida my depression got so bad that even suicide was a thought in my head. I am not afraid to say that now; if it wasn't for me even admitting it to the right people I may not be here today. I would sit in the bathtub for hours, just sitting there, the water getting colder and contemplating what I should do? And I wasn't thinking housework or walks either. People think that it will never happen to them, but until something triggers you, you never know. That is a very dark and cold place to be in and one that I wish was not so easily accessible for people. I am just glad to say that I pulled though that dark period and understand now how and why some end up there. Looking back at how I was acting at this time in my life to, I can totally see how I was must of looked to others, some took it the wrong way, but luckily enough of the right people in my life didn't. Referring to those dark moments, I am utterly amazed that a person can fall so hard and so fast, but I also look now at how lucky I am to be on the other side and see how much some do take their lives and families for granted.

Florida was not my only trip away from home though, or escape after my surgery, I also got a plane ticket to go back to Ontario shortly after getting back from Florida and honestly wasn't sure if I was ever coming back. But something hit me

19

while I was down there and I realized it was time to get my ass in order and straighten up, that I had a husband and two boys at home waiting for their mom to come back. It was great that I have the friends that I do, in both Florida and Ontario, next to my husband waiting for me they were a huge influence in me getting better, or getting me to admit something was seriously wrong. After getting home from Ontario I took myself to counselling, I took it slowly, but did attend my sessions and I am so thankful I did. I think I needed that "opening up" and being honest thing, before I could really move forward. You know I was always the person in school, even back in elementary, that was the bubbly, outgoing and adventurous one and always had a smile on my face, so when I lost that smile, it wasn't me.

Yes, there have been some major changes, friendships lost, people may have different opinions of me now, but I believe and feel that I am in the "right place", that I have nothing more to worry about now, other than to live my life to the fullest. Not all people can handle situations like mine, whether it be friends or family members, sometimes it ruins friendships, relationships, you name it. But life has to go on and you make the best of what you have. Just knowing what my husband and boys had to see and live with, I am so thankful that they didn't give up on me. I love them for still being here. I guess that when we took or vows, "for better or for worse", he was actually paying attention, thank you.

One part of my depression that I felt very "angry" about, was having people tell me, "don't tell this person or that one, they don't need to know". Well you know what, right there sets me off, don't ever tell me I can't say or do something, I am my own person, grown up and will say and do what I wish, of course being very mature about the whole thing, but don't insult my decisions.

They are my choices to make. One very positive figure in my life and who knew about my whole depression ordeal was my grandfather, Grampy, who passed away a few years ago in England. If I needed to talk to someone, I just picked up the phone and dialled his number. I loved that he was always there to answer. Even though we lived thousands of miles from one another we were very close. I still have letters that he wrote me and tend to look at them once in a while. He was so good when it came to anything I did or wanted to do, he never second guessed my choices or put me lower than anyone else, which is what I loved so much about him and still do. In one of his very last letters to me he said, "always do whatever you enjoy doing, lots of love Gramps". My Grampy always knew how I was feeling and what I was going through, I told him everything. More things than I would ever tell my own parents, I am sure they will take that the wrong way, but I don't mean it in a negative way, we were just very close, and it was the kind of relationship you wish you could have with all of your family members, but that usually doesn't happen. Well it took about a year and a half for me to get over the depression, with help from family, friends, counsellors and myself making the effort, it has all worked out in the end. Now I seem to be on the other end of things, I am here now trying to give support, encouragement and help to those going through exactly what I went through. I want to remind people in that predicament to never feel like you can't ask for help or that it is a hopeless trail to go down. There is always a path that can get you in the right place.

Just talking about my Grandfather reminded me of a very interesting experience on one of my trips to Liverpool, England; it was a couple years after my surgery. One of my uncles took me to a museum down by the docks and interesting enough there was a huge display on Epilepsy. It defiantly was not a positive outlook on epilepsy though, but a very disturbing one. It showed that back in the 1700's to late 1800's those with epilepsy, or who had seizures were locked up in jail like buildings. They were thought to be possessed, evil and should not be in contact with others. My first thought was obviously, "how sick were people back than?" and I wasn't meaning those who had seizures. No wonder depression was big, with those who were having seizures, they were locked up. I am not sure how I would of reacted back than, obviously if I did live back in those days and were to of retaliated against the treatment I would have been seen as possessed to. I am so glad that times have changed and people can look at different disorders now with open eyes.

The two medications that I was on and for a very long period of time were Topamax and Tegretol. I found some extremely interesting reading on both of them when it came to side effects. Some of these were dead on with how I felt or experienced. Please note though that this is **MY** experience and I am definitely not suggesting that someone does not take a particular drug or medication. In regards to Tegretol (Carbamazepine) it says at you shouldn't take this medicine if you have a history of bone marrow suppression or if you are allergic to an antidepressant and it also stated that a person may have thoughts about suicide while taking this medication. Interesting! I think that would have been a good point to have known before hand, but again, that doesn't mean everyone who takes these meds all go through the same feelings and side affects. Another logical point is call your doctor at once if you have any new or worsening symptoms such as: mood or behavior changes, depression, anxiety, or if you feel agitated, hostile, restless or hyperactive. Tegretol is also in a group of drugs called anticonvulsants, which works by decreasing nerve impulses that cause seizures and pain it is also used to treat bipolar disorder. Now as far as Topamax goes, it can cause some people to have a sudden change in vision and pain around or behind the eyes, also, some experience mood or behavior changes, depression, anxiety, restless, hyperactive or have thoughts about suicide or hurting yourself, just like the Tegretol. Wow, after reading all of this information, I am curious to know, if maybe I might not have been where I was had I known what some of the effects were or could be. Maybe I would have jumped on the wagon for treatment or help sooner than later. I suppose being on the other end of things now I am just grateful to be where I am. Seizure free and drug free.

I have to admit to that I would never have chosen not to take any meds for my seizures, so in the big picture I am glad I did.

After a year of being seizure free from the surgery I was "slowly" weaned off the Tegretol and Topamax, I was ecstatic about not having to take pills, and 7 of them, every day. It was a slow process, but looking back at it now it actually flew by. I was hoping for some extreme side affects, preferably one being weight loss but for some reason that was the opposite of what happened to me. I actually gained 30 lbs when I was off all 7 pills. Of course I was pleased to be seizure free and done with all the meds, but what a depressing blow that was. I took it all in stride though, knowing that I may have to stay on at least one or two pills depending on how my body reacted to being "drug free" so I called it. But other than the weight gain I think I did pretty well. I was completely off the meds and it felt great, that meant not running up to the pharmacy every couple of weeks to get refills or remembering to even just take the pills. I was done with them! One hard part of the whole seizure free part of it was taking off my medi bracelet, I wore that 24/7, and it was like a permanent fixture on me. The day I removed it and put it in my jewellery box was the day I realized that this was a new beginning, a new start to whatever I had in front of me. Of course when rummaging for earrings or other jewellery I come across it and it does take me back, which I feel, is a good thing. I don't want to forget what I went through, I am going to use that experience to build on my life now and I am going to make it a good one. I am almost 40 years old, been seizure free since my surgery and have never stopped trying to help others in my community through volunteering. My one great accomplishment though is being elected on as Vice President for the Edmonton Epilepsy Association and there are certain people in that organization that know I am thankful to them for believing in me.

I originally started out volunteering on smaller boards with the EEA and made my way up to the Board of Directors, getting involved with the EEA helped my depression; it showed me that I have potential and also that I have what it takes to be a model person for those in need, at least that's how I see myself. I also never stopped doing things that I wanted to do through my years with seizures. I have been a board member with a local RCMP Advisory Board for almost 10 years, even while attending board meetings I had the occasional seizure, fortunately they were always mild ones, petit mal as I still call them. It was nice having board members so supportive with me, if I new I was going into a seizure, having an aura, I usually would let one of the members know, she was awesome to, thanks for not making such a big issue out of a small seizure at those meetings. It normally would take me a few minutes to get back into things, as I do the minutes for all the meetings, I would have to concentrate even harder, as my brain seemed to be in slow motion at times, especially after a seizure.

I have only missed 2 or 3 RCMP board meetings in nine years, and those were because of holidays never because of my seizures. Even after my surgery in December, I attended the January meeting, with my bandana on and pen and paper ready to go. Of course my minutes were a bit simpler than the previous ones, but after a few months my brain seemed to get right back into the groove of things. I am thinking of taking a short break from volunteering on boards, so I can spend more time at home with my kids, especially Nathan who is almost two now, but it will be a short break. Just referring back to my depression after the surgery, I am so thankful that there were board members who noticed the change in me to. I was normally the bubbly outspoken one and when my depression hit I wasn't the same, that wasn't me sitting at the table, quiet and keeping to myself. This was all around the same time that I went to Florida, maybe a few weeks prior. Again, having certain people notice that I was not right was probably the best thing that ever happened to me. I stayed back after one of the board meetings to talk with a couple of the members and from there I started to realize that I needed a way out; I needed to admit something was wrong. I know that I keep thanking people throughout this story, but it is so true that I owe so many people thanks and I just want them to know how much I do appreciate everything that has been done for me. Just remember, don't ever feel controlled by your seizures and don't ever think any less of yourself for needing help from others. Ask questions and make sure you get the answers you are looking for.

5

Sex
and
Seizures

What took you so long to turn to this page?

Sex, Sex, Sex.....I bet a few of you reading my story actually jumped to this chapter first before even reading the introductory page or maybe you didn't even finish reading the table of contents. Don't worry; I won't tell anyone, it is just funny that people seem to get very intrigued when a title or heading has the word "sex" in it. Well I am not going to turn this into an adult related chapter, that will be my next book, but I just wanted to talk a bit about sex and seizures. I personally never even considered or thought that having sex could trigger me to have a seizure, but apparently it can occasionally happen. Sex and Seizures....Sex, what sex! That is how my husband would have commented to that. Women are difficult enough to live with, but throw in a few obstacles, like seizures and wow we can be like living with a brick wall.

In 2009 I had a fabulous time helping out at the Sex and Seizures Forum at the Glenrose Hospital in Edmonton, Alberta. Our speakers were wonderful, the information they had for the audience in regards to Seizures and Sex was so informative. There were questions and comments that I really never thought of before. Questions came from individuals who have Epilepsy, parents who have grown children with Epilepsy and from medical workers, care workers and friends. After the speakers were done I had the privilege of sitting on the question panel with them, what a fabulous experience.

A couple of the questions that I answered were.....

Have you ever had a seizure during sex?

Wow, I thought, that was a good one right of the bat!!! I honestly can say, NO, I am 99% sure I didn't! I did say to the audience though, "let me call my husband and ask him", I got a good laugh out of that. You know that is something throughout my whole life with seizures that I really never thought of... the "what if's" during sex...hmmmm now it seems kind of interesting to think about.

Did the medication you were on affect your sex drive (want for sex)?

That is a **YES**, I found different medications to be very disruptive when it came to Sex, I am very honest with my answers when people ask me anything, and I must say that when I was on Topomax and Tegretol together my sex drive was at its lowest. I must add to that I am SO HAPPY to be 100% off of all meds now! I am sure my husband is as well!!!

Sex and seizures doesn't always go smoothly together, speaking from my own experiences. I found that different meds I was on lowered my sex drive immensely. Sometimes it seemed to "cut me off", sort of speak, or I should say "cut my husband off". I never really looked into reasons for it, I don't think I even asked my doctors why, but since being off all my meds and researching reasons for the change, it all seems to make sense now. I did find an amazing article on Hormones and Seizures, which answered a lot of my questions. Interesting enough there is a dynamic relationship between brain function, hormones and seizures. It has been shown that seizure discharges in certain brain areas can alter the output of hormones from the brain and sex hormones can influence how the brain works. I know I found that during my menstrual cycles (periods) I would tend to have more seizures than when I was not menstruating. Estrogen has been shown to increase seizure activity, while progesterone can have anti-seizure effects. Seizures that are most likely to be affected by hormonal changes are partial seizures, that involve the temporal or frontal lobes of the brain. I tended to have a lot of partial seizures, again during my period. It also said that some seizure medicines can lower your mood, sex drive or cause physical changes that make intercourse painful or less pleasurable. Even throughout my chats on my Epilepsy Support Group site, I recall several conversations in regards to others asking "Why do I have no sex drive?" Why does it hurt?" "Will this ever pass?", "Are my meds causing all of this?" Again, I am not a medical professional, so my answers are from experience and I think that asking others that have gone through the same ordeals is the best way to get answers and support.

Sometimes I find experience is more credible than education, but remember that is **MY** opinion. Don't always think you can solve things on your own and if your doctor isn't an option, than find a support group or health line. Sometimes seizures and sex don't always mix well together, but that doesn't mean for everyone, we are all different in our own ways. There are some great epilepsy websites that talk about sex and seizures, how it affects people differently and also the same.

I have included a few of my favorite websites in this book, take a look through them and maybe you will find what you are looking for, I know I did!

6

Different places where I had seizures Auras

Different places where I have had seizures or auras...

Some people probably never really think twice about where they actually have had a seizure but for me I think I have kept track of pretty much every one of them, especially if they were in awkward, odd or dangerous places. Even remembering an aura coming on in these kinds of places is still tattooed in my mind. These are some of the places, spots or areas that I had auras come on or full blown seizures come about......

- the chair at the dentist office while him working on my teeth
- carrying a coffee down a set of concrete stairs, luckily I was at the bottom stair and had a friend with me who wa able to grab my coffee (and me)
- ordering dinner in a restaurant

- in the bathtub
- getting my hair cut
- boiling water on my gas stove at home
- in the passenger seat of our car, that happened several times…..
- walking in the wooded park by my house
- at work, when I worked at the medical centre
- I even had one or two while at boxing, no I wasn't sparring at the time
- during a soccer game
- and even at the odd board meeting

I suppose my point here is to let people know that someone with epilepsy or that has seizures can still live life like everyone else does; we just might need to take a little extra caution or "mini breaks' I liked to call them to recuperate from a seizure. Just remember safety is number one.

Auras

Auras vary between different people. Yours may happen right before a seizure or several minutes to hours earlier. Common warning signs right before seizures are changes in bodily sensations, changes in your ability to interact with things happening outside of you, and changes in how familiar the outside world seems to you as well. Other warning signs that may happen hours before a seizure are depression, irritability, sleep disruption, nausea, and headache. I always seemed to have an aura before a seizure up until a few months before my surgery; than my seizures would come on so sudden that I didn't have time to "prepare" for one. My auras generally gave me at least a 20 second warning, usually, that way I was able to sit down or get in a safer position depending where I was at the time. An aura to me was like closing my eyes and having a zillion things go through my head at once, it was a very bizarre experience and would explain the feelings of nausea and headaches after the seizure.

I have chatted with several people on line that explain their aura's in almost the exact same way, lights flashing, zillions of things passing by and light headedness. I actually do remember the auras that I had, at least most of them. It was the seizure afterwards that I can't recall at all. One aura that seems to stick in my head is one I had a few weeks before my surgery. I was making dinner in the kitchen, using our gas stove and I was boiling water to make spaghetti. I remember stirring the wooden spoon in circles when that sensation hit me. Shit, I thought, not again. I remember pausing, thinking maybe it will just pass by, as some auras tended to, but not this one. I must have stepped back slightly from the stove and my husband was sitting at the table close by, but he didn't even have time to get out of his chair. I fell like a brick to the floor; I am so lucky that I didn't fall towards the stove with the gas burner on and the water boiling. After that I don't remember anything till I was done having the seizure and it was a big one. Closer to my surgery the seizures were getting so intense, lasting longer and I was having bruises and bumps from my falls, which I can't remember happening that often before. I had a black eye and huge bump on my head, but I got though it. I told myself, only a little bit longer and I go for my surgery. So when I was done the seizure and caught my breath I went back to finishing making dinner. I never said I can't do this or that because of my seizures, it was part of me and I dealt with it.

Another aura that I remember having, but don't recall the seizure was when we lived in Calgary and Richard and I were out for dinner, with Mathew 2 years old at the time. I remember having the sensation that an aura was coming on, but than I don't recall the seizure. It was a partial one, but the strange reaction I had was that I was nodding my head and body back and forth and apparently ordering everything and anything that was on the menu, my poor husband. Eventually I came trough, realizing I had just had a seizure, but decided, yep it is over, let's try ordering again. I am so happy that my days of aura's and having to prepare myself for whatever kind of seizure was about to occur, is over with.

7

Facts
History, Types of Seizures and Medications
and
Did you know?

Myths and Facts about Epilepsy

Here are a few that I thought were quite interesting.......

MYTHS

- Epilepsy is contagious. **(I have always laughed at that one)**
- You can swallow your tongue.
- People with Epilepsy can't work. **(I have ALWAYS worked)**
- People with Epilepsy look different.
- Epilepsy is a mental illness.

FACTS

- The word Epilepsy comes from the Greek word "Seizure".
- Most seizure disorders can be controlled partly or completely by:
  - » Anti-convulsive medication
  - » Surgery
  - » Diet
- Some of the causes are:
  - » Genetic
  - » Brain injury
  - » Developmental disorder
  - » Trauma
  - » Stroke
  - » Infection

History of Epilepsy

400 B.C.

A Greek physician wrote the first book on epilepsy!

1912

In 1912, two independent teams of chemists created Phenobarbital under the name of Luminal. Phenobarbital is the oldest AED in common clinical use.

1929

A German Psychiatrist named Hans Berger announced to the world that it was possible to record electric currents generated on the brain, without opening the skull, and to depict them graphically onto a strip of paper. Berger named this new form of recording as the Electroencephalogram (EEG).

Different types of Seizures

(these are just a few)

I still use the "old" terms myself, Petit Mal and Grand Mal!

Primary Generalized Seizures

- Absence seizures
- Atypical absence seizures
- Myoclonic seizures
- Atonic seizures
- Tonic seizures
- Clonic seizures
- Tonic-clonic seizures

Partial Seizures

- Simple partial seizures
- Complex partial seizures
- Secondarily generalized seizures

"The Brain"
DID YOU KNOW?

- Approximately 0.6% of the Canadian population has epilepsy.
- Each day in Canada, an average of 42 people learn that they have epilepsy.
- In 50 - 60% of cases, the cause of epilepsy is unknown.
- Epilepsy is a disorder, not a disease.
- The major form of treatment is long-term drug therapy.
- Brain surgery is recommended only when medication fails and when the seizures are confined to one area of the brain where brain tissue can be safely removed without damaging personality or function.
- The oldest detailed account of epilepsy is on a Babylonian tablet in the British Museum. This is a chapter from a Babylonian textbook of medicine comprising 40 tablets dating as far back as at least 2000 BC.
- Your brain is the most **energy consuming** part of your body.
- Your brain contains about **100 billion neurons.**
- The human brain is about **75% water.**
- The weight of an average brain is about 3lbs.

Different types of Seizure Medications

The following are currently approved in certain countries and the highlighted ones are those that I have used or tried!

Banzel	Luminal
Carbamazepine	Lyrica
Carbatrol®	Mysoline®
Clobazam	Neurontin®
Clonazepam	Oxcarbazepine
Depakene®	**Phenobarbital**
Depakote®	Phenytek®
Depakote ER®	Phenytoin
Diastat	Primidone
Dilantin®	Rufinamide
Ethosuximide	Sabril
Felbatol®	**Tegretol®**
Felbamate	Tegretol XR®
Frisium	Tiagabine
Gabapentin	**Topamax®**
Gabitril®	Topiramate
Inovelon®	Trileptal®
Keppra®	Valproic Acid
Keppra XR™	Vimpat
Klonopin	Zarontin®
Lamictal®	Zonegran®
Lamotrigine	Zonisamide and Levetiracetam

8

Epilepsy Websites

Logging onto Epilepsy websites is a great way to find support groups, have questions answered and to educate yourself on Epilepsy itself!

Websites

Here are some Epilepsy Websites that provide incredible information, Support Groups in your area, comments and experiences others have dealt with in regards to Epilepsy!

Please check them out!

- www.edmontonepilepsy.org (my favorite)
- www.epilepsyalliance.org
- www.epilepsymatters.com
- www.epilepsy.ca
- www.efa.org
- www.epilepsy.org.uk
- www.medicalert.ca
- www.epilepsy.com
- www.healthywomen.org

There are so many different sites to go on and they are **ALL** very informative and educational, I think that everyone should take the time to check out one or two, educate your own brain!

My On-line Epilepsy Support Group

Here are a few of the emails received on my Life After Brain Surgery group that I have on FACEBOOK.

Check out my support group there are over 120 fantastic people on there!!

April 09

Thanx for that Ann...

Kind words of encouragement, but, as you know, it's a VERY hard decision to make and has taken over my mind completely; got to weigh up the pros and cons I suppose and then decide.

> Take care
>
> Jon
>
> (Plymouth)

April 09

Some people get a great reduction in their Seizures; I guess I am one of those people. I can't Complain, at least I have a reduction in my seizures. Congrats to everyone who is seizure Free.

> Leah
>
> (Oregon, USA)

April 09

I hope everyone the best on there surgery. I had surgery May 22nd 2008. Since that date I haven't had a seizure. Yay! It will be a year next month. I had a left temporal Lobe Lobectomy. Now waiting on the paperwork to say it is ok to get my license, then going to school to help others with the same condition as us.

Ashley

(Florida, USA)

∽◦◦◦

April 09

Hi everyone

Had a right temporal lobectomy at the Walton Centre in Liverpool in January. Still a bit knackered but so far so good. No seizures, just a couple of anxiety attacks in place of them and horrendous depression. Hoping it will go! Take care all xxx

Helen

(England)

∽◦◦◦

March 09

Thank you for the information Ann.

Take care

Mike

(NB, Canada)

∽◦◦◦

March 09

I am now SEIZURE FREE since last Christmas and I am about to apply for my provisional driving license. I am also currently a volunteer in a local NHS hospital and I am hopefully going to do my second degree studying Diagnostic Radiography (Interview on the 14th Jan)

The Surgery was certainly SUCCESSFULL and I never look back!

Adam
(England)

Feb 09

Thanks so much your responses Ann, Mike and Stacey! I have heard some really mixed things about all of this. I am concerned that if I do go through with this than it may not work, and if it does, will it work only a short time. That is a long time to be away from your family and your life to only find yourself back on the medication. Were you guys awake during the surgery? Can you tell me where you had it done and the pros and cons? I have lots of questions and really want to be informed before I make a decision like this one. I was also wondering about the risks and the recovery. Thanks!

Sarah
(USA)

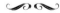

Feb 09

Great to hear success stories here. Thank you all for sharing them with us.

I am writing about my sister's surgery again. She had the surgery on 20th of January. No seizures, no auras since then. I hope she will never have one again.

Mehmet
(Italy)

Jan 09

I just wanted to say by reading everyone stories. I hope you all the best. I had seizures since age 3 now I am 27. I decided to have the brain surgery (left temporal lobe) on May 22nd 2008. Since then I haven't had a seizure. I can say I feel so free and happy. Now planning school and to get my license. I can't wait. If anyone wants to chat or needs someone to talk to I am here. Take care

Ashley
(Florida, USA)

Jan 09

Thank you, all for the talk .I get to go see my doctor in 2 days, the more things I hear from other people, the more I can smile to know I am not alone

Mike
(NB, Canada)

Jan 09

Hi My name is Narelle I am 35 and had left Temporal Lobe surgery on August 25th 1997 it was the best thing I ever did I am now seizure free have not had a seizure for 11 years and now have my drivers license and have moved out into my own unit would love to talk to other people who have had it done

Narelle
(Australia)

Nov 08

Hey there all,

What a great Group....wish it was around when I was younger. Well, I was diagnosed when I was 9 and lived with having petit seizures for 10 years; during that time medication changes and alterations-living with the side effects and EEG's. However when I was 14/15 and started going to the neurologist and he explained brain surgery maybe an option- I was eager to find out more, but he wanted to do some more med trials. Finally we began the pre surgery testing, EEG's MRI, WADA and the 24hr EEG (25days) which took about 2-3 years due to waiting lists but I was a successful canadate for surgery; in May '98 came out a new person; was on meds for 2 or 3 years after however was seizure free and now been off meds since and seizure free. I have accomplished things that I would have never thought of. So...joined this group to provide support and encourage for other; I'm here to chat, listen and have a laugh. hope to be in touch!

Laura
(Toronto, Ontario)

Nov 08

Thanks for the site I am sure it will help a lot of people, it's helped me already, now I don't feel that alone. Xxx

Zoe

(England)

❧

Oct 08

Hi Ann, Thank you for making this group to share experiences about epileptic surgery!

Mehmet

(Italy)

❧

June 08

Thanks Ann. I just am hoping the seizure was a warning sign of too much stress. My doc has been supportive in agreeing to see what happens without the meds. I am investigating some alternative therapies in the meantime.

Melanie

(Calgary, Alberta)

❧

March 08

Wow... I never even knew there was such a group! I had a right Temporal Lobectomy back in 1993 in University Hospital - London, Ontario, Canada.

Seems to have worked wonders! I'm totally off meds and haven't had any seizures since! I even drive a school bus now! Was epileptic from age 1½ until the surgery at age 16. Childhood was awful!! It was like a whole new life after the surgery!

Jonathan
(Windsor, Ontario)

June 07

Hi Ann! Thank you for starting this group. I think we all need each other so we can share our stories and not feel alone. This planet can feel quite lonely sometimes. Lets all get together and help support each other! What an awesome name for a group! Thanks for reaching out.

Trina
(USA)

Those were just a few of the hundreds of emails received in my Epilepsy Support Group. As of today I have over 105 people that have joined my site, what an awesome feeling it is to know I am reaching out to that many, and from everywhere to. It is wonderful to hear from others that live on the other side of the world that are going through or have gone through the same experiences. There are people from Turkey, UK, USA, Canada, Hong Kong and many other places. To me it is a site that can give hope to those to that are just beginning a journey, maybe they are just getting prepared for surgery or new meds; nevertheless, it is great to be able to share with others. Keep up the emails everyone!

In conclusion, to my life with epilepsy, I am going to share with you some of my poems and a couple articles that I had written about my experience with the surgery that cured me 110%! If someone was to ask me right here right now, "would you do this all again?" I would have a huge grin on my face and say **"Damn right I would!"** Life is one of those things that you can't always have guarantees on all the time, you take what you are given and you make the best of what you have, don't always settle for less or think you can't reach the inevitable; it is possible, look at me!

9

Poems,
Photos and Painting
By
Ann Gillie

**The poems with an * beside them are ones
I had published since my surgery.**

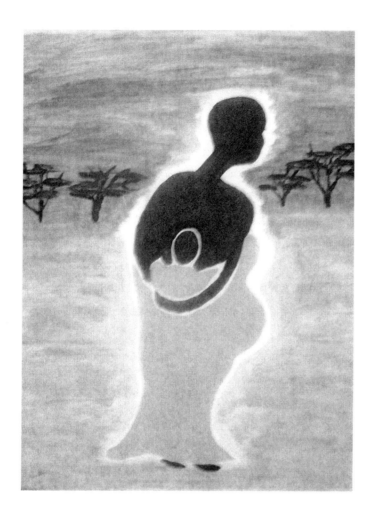

"Expectant mother walking with her small child"

This was my first painting that I did shortly after my surgery. I am not sure what inspired me to paint this, but when I was done it left me with such a positive feeling that I continued to paint and a few years later I did have another son!

The Fly Fisher

Spring creeks rise from chalk beds
The mist lies low
Amongst the brush and trees

On English streams
And rippled lakes
Fly and fish become one

A tradition continues
As the sun awakes from its sleep
Providing a distinctive glow

A true fisherman will say
How one plays the game
Is more important than his catch

Summer at the Lake

Speeding boats
Tubes and skis
Rippling water
Lakes and trees
Seagulls squawking
Sandy beach
Suntan oil
My retreat

Cobblestone Roads

The roundish smooth stone
Patched with color
Joined the streets around
Carriages with horses sat
While the tower clock rang aloud
People shoes sounded like thunder
As they crossed the roads around
These cobblestone roads
Have more character
Than any pavement could wish to have

Tea with the Queen *

My holiday takes me overseas
I am getting away for two to three weeks
No husband or children
What will I do
Maybe visit the Queen
Or fight knights between brews
I get off the plane
Feeling happy and free
Wine in the air
Kicks in rather intensely
My luggage is gathered and I hop in a cab
Off to the palace I say to the lad
He heads for the city
On the wrong side of the road
I forgot here in England
They drive opposite from home
As we approached the palace
The cab driver said
Have you ever met royalty
Or seen the queen sort her gems
I shook my head
And gathered my things
Stood in line at the big tourist gate
I paid my money and was last to go in
My luggage was placed in a very large bin
I made my way down a long corridor
But accidentally went through a wrong brass door
Who was sitting in a large swivel chair

But the Queen herself eating a chocolate éclair
She noticed my accent and asked me to stay
She ordered us tea and we discussed Canada all day
Tea with the Queen was a wonderful day
Every tourist should do it
When touring her domain
Just remember to go through the wrong brass door
Take her chocolate éclairs
Enough for two
Or more

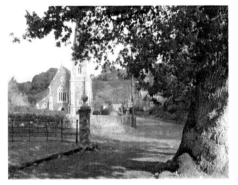

Clearwell, England

Wealth of the Homeless *

With quivering hands
And motionless eyes
They lay in the darkness of life

No laughter or joy
No comfort or hope
They depend on their inner light

Hands held out in shame and guilt
They beg on others
For pennies and dimes

With little hope of reaching high
They fall to darkness
And see no blue sky

No money, jewels or diamond rings
Just coats on their backs
And hearts left in the rain

In sheltered fear
And times of pain
The wealth of living
Is still their highest gain

Driftwood

Along the rough and sandy shore
The dry rugged driftwood lay
I lean against it comfortably
Look around, I am alone
The peaceful mood is divine
I could only wish to live like this
Every day so calm
The waves smashing against the rocks
Is the only sound
The driftwood that I have found
Has lead me to believe
That nature can capture a person's heart
And lead them to their dreams

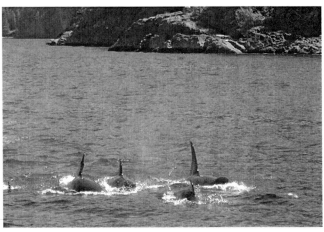

Family of Orcas, Telegraph Cove, Vancouver Island

Life

Pedals falling
Towards the ground
Wind flowing
Through the grass
Birds singing
In the sky
Clouds hovering
From high above
Trees standing
In the forest
Fish swimming
Through the waters
Children playing
On the sidewalks
People live
Day to day
Life is
But many things

Ghosts in the Kitchen

Strange noises in the background
Startle me most days
I hear clatter in the kitchen
And hazy voices you could say
Some days I smell baking
Hear whispers through the walls
Women giggling at my table
And odd noises in the hall

The stories I have been told
Have lead me to believe
That ghosts live in my kitchen
And don't intend to leave
Maybe they grew up here
And maybe they feel safe
I suppose they bring no harm to me
And I do hear them say grace

Ghosts in my kitchen
Is not that big deal
Maybe in my future
I will be joining them for a meal
So if the ghosts in my kitchen
Want to spend their days with me
They need to use their manners
And keep their noises down at tea

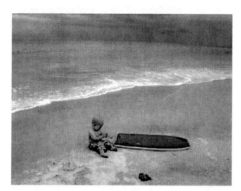

New Smyrna Beach, Florida

Birth

Love and aching
Pain and desire
Screaming
Comfort
Teardrops and joy
Mood swings and tempers
Hugs and kisses
Pushes and pulls
What we go through
What we accomplish
Tap yourself on the back
Listen to that cry
You made that
Love
Joy
That baby

Doubt

He deems uncertain
With suspension at hand
Who to question
Who's the suspect
Can we trust
Or make a stand
Who can pass judgment
Opinions can be cruel
The world has so much doubt
Is there room for equal rule

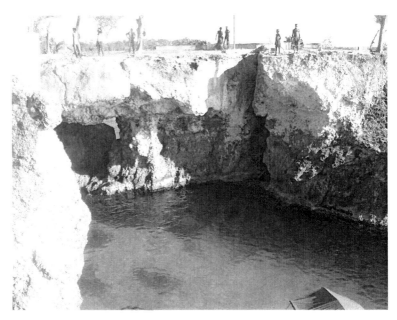

Negril, Jamaica

One Tree

Thousands stand
Together in silence
Leaves falling
To the ground
Nests hidden
Among the branches
Acorns mix
Within the tall grass
Sap trickles
Along the bark
Woodpeckers
Stamp their names aloud
One tree
A large forest
One tree
Seems to always stand out

School Bus

Black yellow
Six big wheels
Flashing lights
Doors of steel
School bags scattered
Under the seats
Noisy kids
Tots to teens
One brave driver
Squeaky seats
We're at school
You hear shuffling feet
The big door opens
Kids get out
Another day starting
See yourself out

Willow Tree *

The porch creeps as I step across
The wood is chipping on the edges
Weeds growing up through the cracks
Boarded windows rusty nails
The tales that could be told
What mysteries lie beneath these boards
I walk around the back
The water pump stands alone
The barn long gone
Two lovely graves in the distance
A willow tree with two carved names
The same as on the graves
A flowing stream right beside
Sets the mood to humble
It takes you back eighty years
You wonder how life was than
So simple
Did that porch creek
How it must have been
To live by that willow tree

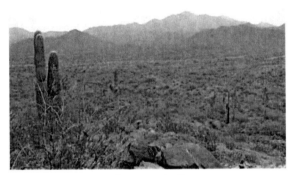

Goodyear, Arizona

Haiku Poems

Creeks gently flowing
Encouraging all which is around
Beauty can be so simple

The pacific ocean
Situated to make peace
Pacifying and calm

Misty sky set above
Rain gently begins to fall
Sets the mood humble

A mothers arms
Is like a touch of magic
Gracefully uplifting

Flocking seagulls dance
Waves interweave with another
Footprints in the sand

That which is positive
Can shine light on another
Provide needed strength

Fog, a dense vapor
Near the surface of land
Or mental confusion *

Imagination
Creativity all people need
Expand their horizons

Simplicity and grace
Our life's reasons for living
Which nature provides

As seasons do change
Memories tagging along
Another year slips by

Footprints in the sand
Get washed away by water
But can be made again

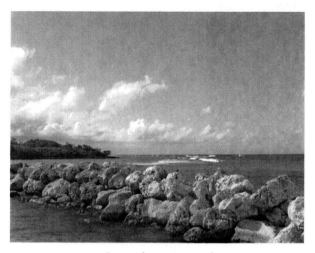

Ocho Rios, Jamaica

Here are 2 stories about my "Epilepsy" experience that were written in 2006 and 2007!

**Edmonton Epilepsy News Release and an article published
in *Your Health Magazine***

FOR IMMEDIATE RELEASE – March 1, 2006

March is Epilepsy Awareness Month
Seizure-Free After Epilepsy Surgery: One Woman Tells Her Story

Ann Gillie was diagnosed with both convulsive and non-convulsive seizures at two years of age. It took several years for doctors to find the right combination of medications that made her seizure free from 9 to 20 years of age, however, they did return in the summer of 1990.

In spite of remaining active, volunteering for local organizations and being the mother of 2 very active boys, Ann struggled with her seizures. The seizures interfered with her ability to drive as well as day to day activities. For example, if Ann had a seizure she would lose touch with her surrounding and could be tired afterwards for an hour. Ann tried many different medications with limited effect.

After extensive testing, it was determined that Ann was a surgical candidate that could potentially cure her of her epilepsy. On December 03, 2002, Ann underwent a selective amygdalohippocampectomy (a big word for a relatively small area of the brain) and has been seizure free since. Initially, Ann struggled with some depression that was related to the surgery; however she continued to be active working and volunteering.

It has been over three years since Ann's surgery and she has been seizure free and off of all her medications. Ann attributes much of her success to her "husband and true friends who stick by her side through ups and downs".

Today, Ann's goal is to "help others, to be able to speak on the topic of epilepsy and on the effects experienced after surgery".

Edmonton Epilepsy Association

This is my story that was published in the March/April 2007 issue; there are a lot of repeated events and topics that have already been spoken about in this book, but it was a story that I was very proud of having published and wanted to add it in as a closure to my book. I also want to add that after my surgery I had 4 poems published, they are the ones in this book with the * beside them as I previously mentioned.

Take Care and thank you for taking the time to read about what I had to say!

Ann

When it came to curing my epilepsy, it turned out that surgery and a little positive thinking were the answer!

My blue and white soccer bag, emblazoned with the crest of a Liverpool team, was packed and sitting by the door for a week before I was admitted to the University of Alberta Hospital. It was December 3, 2002, three weeks before my 33rd birthday. I was determined that this would become an anniversary that my family could celebrate in the years to come. The kids – Mathew, then 8 and Cameron, 4 – were at their grandparents' house. My husband Richard had taken time off to be with me in the hospital and at home after the surgery.

I was about to have a small portion of my brain removed in order to try and put a stop to the epileptic seizures I'd experienced for most of my life. So Richard and I got into the car at six that morning and drove through the pre-dawn snow to the University of Alberta Hospital. I could tell Richard was tense but he still tried to put me at ease. I didn't need to be put at ease

I was giddy and kept up a steady stream of chatter the whole way to the hospital. "Are you ready for this?" Richard asked me. I'd never been so ready. I wasn't scared. I was more excited than I had been on our wedding day. I think I even raised an eyebrow or two at the hospital. I guess brain surgery patients aren't usually so thrilled. But I wanted to put an end to the seizures which were a constant worry. Just two days before my surgery I was cooking dinner when I got an aura. I started to feel sort of detached, or spacey. I reached out and fumbled for the switch to turn off the stove burner. I made it to the living room, sinking to the couch before the seizure started.

My seizures, both petit mal and grand mal, all started with auras that lasted about half a minute. (The seizures themselves were generally less than two minutes.) The auras were warning signs that saved me from hurting myself or someone else, either through falling or dropping something. I could get into a safe position, either onto a bed or floor. If I was with someone, I could warn them. But the auras couldn't tell me if the seizure was going to be a short petit mal or an aggressive grand mal. The seizure I had that day turned out to be a grand mal. Three-quarters of an hour later, I was back to the business of dinner, feeling sore and decidedly wrung out. As I stirred the spaghetti sauce, I wondered if I'd just had my last seizure.

People with epilepsy can live normal lives. It creates obstacles, but you can work around them, especially with the support of family and friends. Epilepsy is a brain condition characterized by recurrent seizures. Approximately 10% of Canadians will experience at least one seizure in their lifetime, but about 1 in 100 have epilepsy. That means there are 15,000 people in Edmonton and Northern Alberta with the disorder and 39 million people worldwide.

In 400 BC, the Greek physician Hippocrates wrote the first description of epilepsy and considered it a physical disorder. But people still thought epilepsy was a curse, demonic possession or some kind of prophetic power. It's described in the bible and once was considered the mark of a witch. In the early 1900s the first epilepsy specialists emerged and two independent teams of chemists created Phenobartial, which is the oldest epilepsy medicine in clinical use (it's the first medication I ever took for my seizures). In 1929, German psychiatrist Hans Berger devised a way to record the electric currents generated by the brain and render them graphically into a series of peaks and valleys. This test is the EEG (electroencephalograph), of which I've had several.

There are several types of seizures and a variety of reasons behind them. The EEG allows doctors to see what a seizure looks like on paper. I know what they're like from inside. My husband Richard tells me that when I was in the grip of a petit mal seizure, I nodded my head, made noises with my lips and sometimes rambled, but mostly just made noise without forming sentences. I don't remember these details.

Most of the time I wouldn't fall, and I remained half aware of what went on around me, but I couldn't respond to people. If I felt a seizure coming on while I was at work, I'd sit down and grab the phone, hoping it would be a petit mal and nobody would notice. Once, I was in line at the IGA and I felt an aura. Fortunately it turned into a petit mal. The cashier kept talking to me but I couldn't understand, or answer.

I just kept "searching" for something in my bag, unable to stop until the seizure eased a minute later. The grand mals were far more intense. They would cause me to convulse, shaking. My eyes would roll back and I would have to be watched so that I didn't hurt myself on anything around me. The grand mals were exhausting. It would take me a half an hour to get back into what I'd been doing.

There are different treatments for epilepsy, from medications to natural therapy. There always seemed to be drawbacks to my meds: weight gain, loss of sex drive or irritability. For most of my life, medication was my only treatment. I was investigating a naturopathic treatment when I switched doctors and heard about a new surgery. If I was an eligible candidate, it meant I could be medication- and seizure-free.

I was two when my first seizure happened. I don't remember it, but my mom says she was in the kitchen making dinner and my dad was reading the newspaper. My brother Mike, then four years old, ran into the kitchen telling them that I was acting funny in my bed. I'd been sick with a fever and my mom found me shaking; my color was off and my breathing very shallow. My parents were horrified and immediately rushed me to the hospital. I was prescribed Phenobarb several times a day.

My seizures slowed and finally stopped when I was about nine years old. I was taken off meds and was free of epilepsy – inexplicably and happily – for 10 full years. In the summer of 1990 I went on holidays with my mom to Vancouver Island. We were visiting a friend's house in Campbell River when my mom looked over at me and noticed that I was acting funny – staring, muttering and not answering questions. She knew it was a petite mal.

Nobody can say why my seizures stayed away so long, or why they returned, but I was absolutely devastated. Just months before, I had started seeing Richard; I was dreading how this would affect our relationship. I felt embarrassed and worried that at my age, seizures would interfere with everything: my social life, love life – you name it. But Richard took it in stride. He took me to most of my doctor's appointments. He had to, because I lost my driver's license that summer. I was 20 and miserable. Everyday, I'd walk by my car keys hanging at the front door and see my red Nissan Sentra sitting out front of our house.

But we managed to continue living a pretty normal life. I made some adjustments on how far away I worked and how I got there, and I always took my pills. Gradually the seizures lessened and my dosages lowered.

A few years down the road the seizures crept up on me again. Richard and I were married and our first son was born in December, 1994. Doctors told me to keep up with the meds and I was seizure-free during my entire pregnancy. I worried about the effect of the meds on the baby, but Mathew was born healthy with all his fingers and toes.

Not long after he was born, the seizures started again. I was a new mom, but stubborn as ever. I didn't want to be told to be careful with my baby, but I knew I had to be. I changed Mathew on the bed or the floor rather than a change table. I always sat on the floor with him or on furniture in the carpeted living room. I never took him for walks or bathed him (or myself) if I was alone. We had a pretty good routine going.

My son Cameron was born in November 1998, and again my pregnancy was seizure free. But after Cameron was born, the grand mals seemed to increase. My medications were increased to seven pills a day of both Tegretol and Topamax, which I hated because of their side effects. But I had two children at home and needed to control the seizures. Then, in 2002, I decided to change doctors for a fresh approach. My family doctor, Dr. Jeff Moss, referred me to a new neurologist, Dr. Robert Pokroy.

He referred me to the University of Alberta Hospital to see Dr. Donald Gross, who said there were new surgical treatments available for some types of epilepsy. That referral changed my life forever. Dr. Gross sent me for a complex set of tests, called EEG Video

Telemetry Monitoring, to see if they could pinpoint where in my brain the seizures were coming from. They attached about 30 wires to my head. (It wasn't a nice look.) I spent the next eight days in a small room while they recorded my brain patterns. I watched enough DVDs on my laptop to last a lifetime. And I had enough seizures for the neurologists to see where they were coming from.

They told me I had focal ictal onset in the left temporal region. A small region of my brain had been damaged during the high fever I had when I was two. The seizures originated there, making me a candidate for a "left selective amygdalohippocampectomy" to remove the damaged tissue.

I was so excited. My husband and I went to see Dr. Matt Wheatley, a neurosurgeon, who seemed relaxed and confident about the procedure. He really put us at ease. "It's like he was talking about removing a hangnail," Richard joked after we'd left. The eight-hour surgery went off without a hitch and I don't remember much about the following day. Later, they took the bandages off, and it looked even worse than the wires. I had 50 staples in my half-shaved head, but amazingly, nothing hurt. It was nothing a bandana couldn't cover.

My recovery was like my hair – it grew slowly, in stages. For a few days after the surgery I really had to work at walking; it was like I was learning over again. I had a therapist, and we would walk as far as the nurse's desk before we went back to my room.

My best friend of 30 years, Jillian, who lives in Florida, called me several times. Her calls were good for me, because I had to walk to the phone by the nurses' desk.

I also had to work on my memory skills. Various Capital Health therapists worked with me on my memory and general motor skills for more than a year. But it's been four years since the surgery and I am 100% back to where I was before, if not better. I am finding that I do need to manage my days differently than before; even though my memory is back, I still need reminders. My calendar is full of "to dos" like work hours and appointments.

After the surgery, I fell into a depression that I didn't expect, even though I was warned that it was a common effect of neurosurgery. It was like being on a roller coaster and not knowing if it was going to stop. Some days were normal, but there were dark, stressful days as well.

Gradually, my depression improved. I also started to write poetry shortly after my surgery. It was a new experience for me and was kind of therapeutic, I think. Even through my seizures and after the surgery, I have always remained very active in my community, which has helped me through the healing process. I live in Spruce Grove, work part-time at the Trans Alta Tri Leisure Centre and I'm a teacher's assistant with Parkland County Schools I have been a member of the Spruce Grove RCMP Advisory Board for seven years and even managed to attend a meeting a month after my surgery. A few months after the surgery, I also started an epilepsy support group in Spruce Grove.

In 2005 I joined the Edmonton Epilepsy Association as a volunteer on one of their boards and I had the goal of becoming a director. I am happy to say that in 2005 I became a member of the Board of Directors, partly thanks to the patience of Daphne Quigley, a nurse for Capital Health who let me bombard her with questions about the EEA and supported me before and after my surgery.

Since my surgery and the long recovery, I have not had a single seizure or taken any meds. I feel like a new person – in fact, so much so that Richard and I decided to add to our family, and recently found out that we're expecting our third child. My life was great before surgery, but now it's great and seizure-free. I wouldn't change a thing. - Ann Gillie

Your Health Magazine - Mar/Apr. 2007 Issue

About the author

I was born December 21, 1969 in Toronto, Ontario and at two years old my journey with seizures began. Living almost half of my life with epilepsy was like living in an obstacle course, never knowing which way my day was going to go. In my early years I was involved with everything, soccer, gymnastics, judo and equestrian riding, seizures may of put a yield on things, but having them, never stopped me from doing things I enjoyed. It definitely was a struggle at times, never knowing when a seizure was going to happen or if it was going to be a mild one, as I would refer to them, but I didn't let my seizures control me. For me going for a second opinion changed my life forever and that is one decision that I feel today is the best one I have ever made. Shortly after my surgery I started a local Epilepsy support group, P.A.C.E (Parkland Aiming at Care for Epilepsy) in Spruce Grove, Alberta, and it has lead me to so many new avenues to go down. Presently, I am working on speaking internationally and I know I will do it; I don't give up easily on things I believe in. I am thinking to, that maybe politics should be my next venture! You never know! I can be full of surprises!

Ann Marie Gillie

Acknowledgements

I obtained my information from **Epilepsy.ca**,
Epilepsy Matters, Epilepsy.com and
Edmonton Epilepsy Association website,
as well as my own personal experiences.
Thank You

I appreciate you letting me share my life story,
my opinions and my thoughts with you.
If I even touched just one person with my story
I feel I have accomplished more than I could wish for!

Thank you
Ann Gillie

"Seizures can affect your life, but should never control it!"
Ann

CPSIA information can be obtained at www.ICGtesting.com
Printed in the USA
LVOW07s0549271215

467839LV00003B/154/P